EATING FOR
Happiness

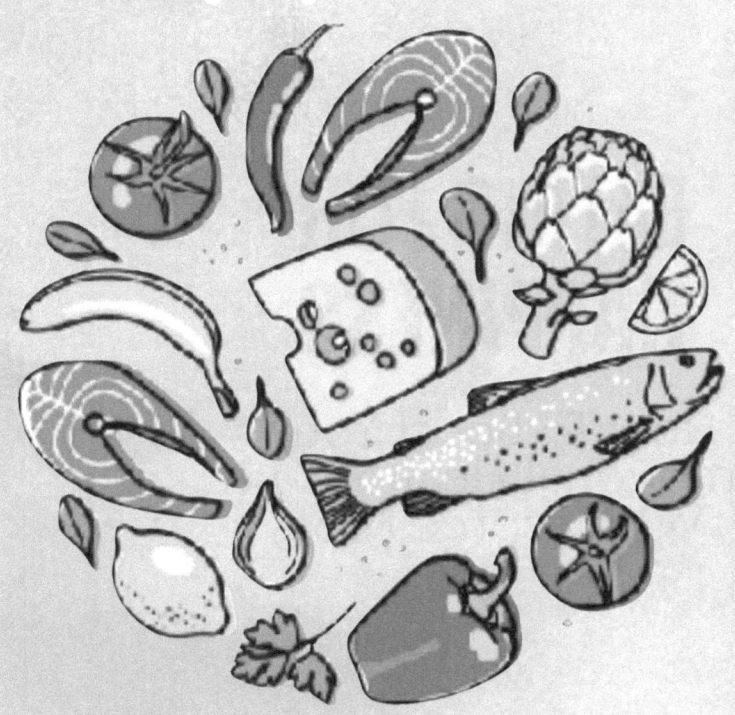

HOW TO BOOST YOUR EMOTIONAL HEALTH WITH WHOLESOME FOOD

EATING FOR
HAPPINESS

How To Boost Your
Emotional Health With
Wholesome Food

TABLE OF CONTENTS

INTRODUCTION

Your diet can affect your health, wellbeing, and happiness. From foods that boost your brain to foods that bring back warm memories, what you put on your plate matters.

Your emotional wellbeing is linked to food.

You may be able to boost your mood with specific diet changes. Although in general, it's important to follow a healthy diet, there are also particular things you can do to ensure you're getting the full benefits from your diet.

What if the pursuit of happiness started with your dinner plate?

By changing what and how you eat, you may be able to influence your mood in a positive way and strengthen your health at the same time.

"Food is for eating, and good food is to be enjoyed. . . I think food is, actually, very beautiful in itself."

- Delia Smith

ELIMINATE OR REDUCE PROCESSED FOODS

The first step to eating for happiness is to eliminate or reduce processed foods. The goal is to cut them completely out of your diet, but this may not be easy right away. Instead, start by reducing the amount of processed foods you eat.

Processed foods tend to have low nutritional value and high levels of sugar.

Research shows that eating large amounts of sugar can affect your brain by shrinking brain cells. This causes your mood to change and reduces your happiness.

If you want to be happy and healthy, it's important to cut down on sugary, processed foods. If you eat much sugar now, you'll want to take this step slowly because sugar is addictive.

Following these strategies will help you reduce the amount of sugar and processed foods you eat:

1. **Read labels.** There are processed foods that are healthier and have less sugar. Although your goal is to cut them out completely from your diet, you can start by focusing on healthier versions of processed foods.

    • Most importantly, **eliminate all processed foods that have artificial sugars or trans fats.**

2. **Learn the different names for sugar.** Sugar can hide under many different names on labels. There are more than 60 different names for sugar used by food manufacturers. Although you may not be able to remember all of them, you can focus on the most common ones and memorize them.

   - Sugar is also called sucrose, corn syrup, high-fructose corn syrup, corn sweetener, barley malt, maltose, dextrose, cane crystals, cane sugar, fructose, maltodextrin and other names.

3. **Designate several days a week to eat without processed foods.** Similar to meatless Mondays or vegetarian Wednesdays, you can create no-processed food

Saturdays or Sundays. This will help you decrease your dependence on processed foods.

- There are also other benefits of these no-processed food days: By setting aside days to be free from all processed foods, you'll also learn to cook from scratch. Plus, you'll find that you're planning healthier meals.

4. **Remember the power of sugar.** Processed food is filled with sugar to influence your taste buds. The reason why manufacturers put sugar in processed foods is that they know it's addictive and powerful.

- It won't be easy to get rid of the sugar in your diet all at once.

However, you can slowly detox from it.

- Sugar doesn't just hurt your waistline. **Too much sugar can negatively affect your brain, mood, and happiness.**

One of the first steps to emotional wellbeing with food is to cut out or reduce processed foods. The high levels of sugar can hurt your brain and affect your mood in a negative and substantial way.

"Research has shown that even small amounts of processed food alter the chemical balance in our brain and cause negative mood swings along with noticeable dips in energy."

- Marilu Henner

FOCUS ON PLANT FOODS

Once you've started to eliminate or reduce processed foods, you'll have more room in your diet for plant foods.

Research shows that a plant-based diet can heighten brain function and uplift your mood.

A plant-based diet also provides your brain with more nutrients such as minerals and vitamins, so you're able to function at the highest levels and find happiness.

There are essential nutrients in plant foods that can increase your happiness.

It's important to be aware of the minerals and vitamins that are naturally found in plant foods, so you can ensure you're getting enough of them.

Consider these important nutrients:

1. **Calcium.** Calcium can be found in a variety of plant-based foods including soy, tofu, broccoli, almonds, seaweed, figs, sesame seeds, and dark, leafy greens.

   - You can get plenty of calcium from plant foods, so you don't need to turn to dairy or meat.

   - **Calcium is important for emotional wellbeing because it affects your nerves and mood.** It can have a calming effect on your nerves.

- In addition to helping build strong bones, calcium is important for lowering blood pressure, encouraging healthy sleep cycles, and fighting anxiety.

2. **Iron.** You may think of meat when you hear iron, but many plant foods also provide high levels of this nutrient.

   - Iron can be found in almonds, dark, leafy greens, beans, legumes, and whole grains.

   - **Iron is important for emotional wellbeing because it helps move oxygen through your body and brain.** This affects your mood and emotional state.

3. **Magnesium.** Magnesium can be found in whole grains, dark, leafy greens, cacao, nuts, seeds, bananas, and sweet potatoes.

- Magnesium is involved in mood regulation.

- It can also positively influence sleep cycles, decrease headaches, decrease migraines, and affect other parts of your body.

4. **Omega-3.** Omega-3 is involved in healthy brain function that has an impact on your moods.

- Omega-3s are found in fish and many plant-based foods. You can add more omega-3s to your diet by eating chia seeds, dark, leafy greens, flax seeds, walnuts, and other seeds.

A plant-based diet can give your body and mind essential nutrients that affect your mood and happiness.

"History has demonstrated that a diet of specific vegan foods, eaten in a specific caloric ratio, will meet all those criteria.

For healing inflammatory bowel diseases, other gut disorders and most other illnesses, I have learned which are the most beneficial foods of all. Those foods comprise what I call the Vegan Healing Diet."

- Dr. David Klein

EAT MORE EGGS

When you're focused on using food to increase your emotional wellbeing, consider the simplicity of eating more eggs.

Eggs are inexpensive and easy to find in most grocery stores. They provide a variety of nutrients that are important for your body and brain, which will naturally boost your energy.

See how an egg can be considered a nutritional powerhouse:

1. **Vitamin D.** Low levels of vitamin D have been linked to depression and mood disorders. Eggs have high levels of this important vitamin.

2. **Folate.** Eggs also have a large amount of folate that affects neurotransmitters in the brain.

3. **Iodine.** Eggs are one of the sources of iodine. Iodine is essential for your thyroid to function properly. It influences your mood. When your thyroid isn't working efficiently, you may experience fatigue, lethargy, depression, and other health issues.

4. **Vitamin B12.** Vitamin B12 can also affect your mood. Low levels of this vitamin are linked to depression, cognitive and thinking issues, and irritability.

5. **Choline.** Plays an important role in brain development and function.

Eggs are versatile, so you can add them to multiple dishes. **Here are a few ways to eat more eggs:**

- They're a popular breakfast option with scrambled, boiled, poached and other variations appearing on multiple menus. You can create your own breakfast favorite by experimenting in the kitchen.

- You can add eggs to soups and casseroles.

- Consider cutting up eggs and putting them in salads. Tuna salad, potato salad, and other versions are easy to make.

- Frittatas and omelettes are also fun ways to eat more eggs.

- Consider using eggs to top sandwiches and toast or mixing them into spreads for your bread.

Whether you make omelettes a regular part of your diet or choose scrambled eggs, the key is to ensure you're getting eggs in your diet. This powerful source of nutrients can positively affect your emotional wellbeing.

"Now that I have a 16-month-old son, my weekend ritual has changed – but it's better than ever. We get up early and go for a walk on one of the hiking trails near my home in Los Angeles, then meet up with friends at a diner. There's nothing better than sipping coffee, eating scrambled eggs, and taking three hours to do it."

- Connie Britton

ADD ANCHOVIES

Anchovies are small, salt-water fish that tend to be sold in brine or salt. They're slender, so you often see multiple fish inside a package at a store.

Although anchovies are sometimes a popular topping for pizza, you may want to add them to your diet in other ways. They're an important and easy-to-find source of nutrients that can boost your happiness.

Learn more about anchovies:

1. **Anchovies contain omega-3.**
   Anchovies have enormous levels of omega-3s packed into a small space. You can get your daily recommended amount by simply

eating this fish. Anchovies have more omega-3s than tuna.

- You already know that omega-3s can influence your mood in a positive way. **Studies show they may have an impact on reducing depression that is mild or moderate.** In addition, they may benefit patients suffering from bipolar disorder.

2. **Get a higher IQ.** Research shows that omega-3s found in anchovies may result in higher IQ levels in children.

- Although a higher IQ isn't a guarantee of happiness, it can make life easier by helping you do better in school and at work. It can affect multiple parts of your life since you'll be less likely to struggle to understand things, so you reduce frustrations that affect your mood.

You can add anchovies to several dishes. **Here are a few ways:**

- Anchovies taste great with pasta dishes. You can cut them into small pieces and mix them with the noodles or simply layer the whole fish on top.

- Anchovies are also good as toppings on top of sandwiches or toast.

- This fish can be added to leafy greens such as Caesar or vegetable salads.

- Anchovies are often used in sauces because of the dramatic flavor. They can be mixed with tomato or cream based sauces.

You can add more anchovies to your diet without affecting your budget. Consider adding them to salads or topping sandwiches with this fish.

"Add anchovies to almost anything, in moderation, and it will taste better."

- Jay McInerney

GET CREATIVE WITH TOMATOES

Tomatoes may already be a part of your diet, but adding more of them may increase your happiness. **There are several mood enhancers naturally found in tomatoes.**

These red treasures can affect your emotional wellbeing, and they're considered a healthy option for dieters.

See how tomatoes can help you:

1. **Tomatoes have lycopene.** Lycopene is responsible for the bright red color you see in tomatoes. However, it also has other uses:

- Lycopene can affect your mood.

- It can prevent inflammation in the body that has been linked to an increased risk of depression.

- Eating more colorful foods can also affect your mood, according to research.

2. **Get a brain boost.** Tomatoes also have folate, vitamin B6, magnesium, and iron. These nutrients can boost your brain and affect your mood. They've been linked to neurotransmitters that affect how you feel.

Tomatoes are one of the easiest plants to add to your diet. **Here are a few ways to eat more tomatoes:**

- Tomatoes are popular in sauces or salsas. From regular tomato sauce to pasta sauce, you can use them to dress up many dishes.

- Fresh tomatoes taste delicious as a part of salads or sandwiches.

- You can add them to juices or smoothies. They blend easily and the seeds don't have to be removed.

- Tomatoes can be baked into casseroles or other dishes.

- They can also be a soup of their own. They make a creamy soup that is perfect for dipping bread.

Tomatoes can boost your mood with their red color and nutrients. They're easy to add to your diet and taste great in many meals.

"You know, when you get your first asparagus, or your first acorn squash, or your first really good tomato of the season, those are the moments that define the cook's year. I get more excited by that than anything else."

- Mario Batali

ADD CHILI PEPPERS

If you're not eating chili peppers, then you're missing out on an important spicy food that can strengthen your emotional wellbeing.

Chili peppers are hot, colorful, and spicy!

They're part of the nightshade family and related to plants such as potatoes and eggplant. However, if you've ever had a chili pepper sauce, then you probably remember the kick it provides to your taste buds.

Stock up on them in the kitchen to elevate your mood!

Chili peppers have many culinary uses:

1. **Chili peppers contain capsaicin.** Capsaicin is a molecule found naturally in chili peppers.

   - Inside your brain, you have receptors that fit the capsaicin molecule. When they fit, your brain releases endorphins that are responsible for making you feel happier and better.

   - This is why many people can't stop eating chili peppers once they get used to the taste. They're benefitting from the release of endorphins and want to keep getting the rush by eating the peppers.

- Endorphins can also calm you.

2. **How to eat more chili peppers.**
   Although it takes time to get used
   to them, you can start with small
   amounts.

   - Chili peppers are popular in
     salsas and sauces.

   - You can use dried versions if you
     don't have access to fresh chili
     peppers, and add them to many
     dishes.

   - A small amount of chili can be
     added to sweet things like
     chocolate for an extra kick.

   - Chili peppers can enhance any
     soup or casserole. They can also

be added to healthy pizzas and low-carbohydrate fries.

- Consider making a chili stew with potatoes, tomatoes, and other vegetables.

- Try the traditional chiles rellenos that are stuffed peppers with sauces on top and other ingredients.

Chili peppers are a spicy diet booster that can positively affect your mood.

"I've got this thing for spicy stuff. Now, if you give me hot chocolate with chili pepper, a book and a bubble bath, I'm a happy girl."

- Shiloh Walker

SPRINKLE MORE BLUEBERRIES

You may enjoy sprinkling blueberries over your cereal or oatmeal in the morning. However, are you aware of how these blue, tiny berries are affecting your emotional wellbeing?

Blueberries can boost your mood and offer other health benefits. They're easy to add to many dishes, so you won't struggle to come up with new recipes. They're also delicious and add a touch of sweetness that won't make you worry about diabetes.

Blueberries can be part of a healthy diet:

1. **Stop cortisol.** Cortisol is a hormone that can increase stress. Fortunately, **blueberries can**

interfere with the process of releasing cortisol, thereby reducing your stress.

2. **Increase anthocyanidins and antioxidants.** Both anthocyanidins and antioxidants are found in high amounts in blueberries.

If you're tired of simply adding blueberries to cereal or oatmeal, consider these other ideas:

- Add blueberries to what you're baking. Scones, muffins, and bread taste better with blueberries.

- Add blueberries to jams or spreads. They're perfect for spreading on crunchy toast or bread. They're also delicious on crackers. Blueberries can be mixed with other berries for a more diverse jam.

- Sprinkle blueberries on top of your salad. They can enhance lettuce.

- Add frozen blueberries to shakes, juices, or smoothies. They make everything blue and tasty.

- Eat them raw as a fun snack instead of chips or pretzels.

- Blueberries are good additions to granola or trail mixes. They can be used as fresh or dried versions.

- Make your breakfast special with blueberry pancakes.

- Consider adding blueberries to your fruit salsa. The combination of these berries with limes and strawberries is delicious.

The impact of blueberries on your emotional wellbeing can't be underestimated. Research shows that these small berries are powerful.

"I may never be happy, but tonight I am content. Nothing more than an empty house, the warm hazy weariness from a day spent setting strawberry runners in the sun, a glass of cool sweet milk, and a shallow dish of blueberries bathed in cream. When one is so tired at the end of a day one must sleep..."

-Sylvia Plath

GO HEAVY ON THE GARLIC

Garlic often gets a bad reputation because it affects your breath. However, as long as you keep toothbrushes and toothpaste nearby, you want to go heavy on the garlic and make it a big part of your diet.

Garlic has multiple health benefits that range from antibacterial to anti-inflammatory properties.

Learn more about garlic:

1. **Garlic contains high levels of chromium.** This nutrient can affect your brain by influencing the production of serotonin. Serotonin is responsible for your mood and how happy you feel. **When there is**

more serotonin being released, you feel happier.

2. **Research shows that garlic can increase your energy and reduce lethargy.** It can also reduce insomnia and anxiety, so you're able to sleep better.

Garlic isn't the easiest food to eat because of its smell and taste. **Here are a few ways:**

- If you can tolerate it raw, chopping garlic into small cloves makes it bite-sized. The addition of honey to raw garlic makes it easier to eat.

- It's easier to add garlic while you're cooking.

- Garlic is a popular addition to pizza crusts and breads. Add it while you're preparing the dough or brush it on at the end.

- Make pasta sauce with garlic.

- Garlic can be added to dips and spreads. It works well with other herbs such as thyme or rosemary.

- Garlic can be part of salad dressings. Minced garlic is easy to add to ranch sauce.

- Consider adding some garlic to your mashed potatoes. They can enhance the taste and make the dish more interesting.

- Blend it into hot sauce.

- Make a unique guacamole by adding garlic instead of cilantro.

The next time you're making pasta sauce, consider going heavy on the garlic. Your body and brain will thank you, and you'll be happier at the end of the night even if you're staring at a sink of dirty dishes.

"My plat de resistance is potato salad with garlic and olive oil which we press from the olives from my trees in the grounds of my home near St Remy de Provence. I have four hectares and take the olives down to the local community press at Maussane les Alpilles. I don't produce big quantities; it is just for the family and friends."

- Jean Reno

TRY PURE MAPLE SYRUP

Although you want to limit sugars on a diet that focuses on happiness, some sweetness is allowed and will help you avoid temptation. Pure maple syrup can add a touch of sweetness in small amounts.

The key is to find pure maple syrup made from the actual trees instead of one that is produced in a laboratory.

Unfortunately, most of the bottles you see in a grocery store aren't pure maple syrup.

- You won't get the health or mood benefits from the artificial syrup.

- The artificial version is made with corn syrup or high fructose syrup instead of coming from a maple tree. Artificial syrup gets its color from caramel dyes.

How do you find pure maple syrup? The key is to read the label. Real and pure products will only have one ingredient: maple syrup. You won't see any added sugars, dyes, preservatives, or other chemicals.

Pure maple syrup has multiple nutrients that can boost your mood:

1. **Manganese.** Important for energy production and antioxidant defenses.

2. **Zinc.** Essential to maintain a healthy immune system.

3. **Riboflavin (Vitamin B2).** Helps the metabolic process.

4. **Calcium.** Strengthens your bones and teeth.

In addition to these minerals, pure maple syrup has **more than 60 antioxidants** that fight cell damage and keep your body healthy. Antioxidants can also affect your mood, since brain cells can be affected by oxidative stress.

How do you use pure maple syrup? The easiest way to use it is to spread it on your pancakes. However, there are other options:

- Use it instead of honey in recipes.

- Add it to baked goods. For example, miniature cheesecakes can be made with this syrup.

- Add it to quinoa.

- Enrich granola or trail mixes. It can also add flavor to energy bars you make at home.

- Consider making fruit kebabs and using maple syrup as a dip instead of caramel or other products.

- Salad dressings and vinaigrettes. You can combine it with lemon or lime and other ingredients such as rice wine vinegar.

Pure maple syrup has health benefits that artificial versions lack. Enjoy adding real maple syrup to your diet!

"The food that's never let me down in life is porridge, especially with milk and maple syrup, which is delicious. Paris isn't a porridge place, but I can buy it in London when I'm there and bring it back with me."

- Marianne Faithfull

INCREASE WHOLE GRAINS

How many whole grain products do you eat every day? The white bread to make toast for breakfast doesn't count, so you may be getting fewer whole grains than you realize. Whole grains are an important part of a healthy diet.

Research shows that whole grains have crucial B vitamins, including B6. Your body and brain need B vitamins for optimal health.

- Studies show that not getting enough B vitamins **increases the risk of depression and anxiety.**

- If you're lacking B vitamins, you may feel irritable or lethargic.

Don't be afraid of carbohydrates. Although you want to limit sugar, complex carbohydrates from whole grains are healthy and important. Your body needs a mix of carbohydrates with other nutrients to function.

- Complex carbs found in whole grains are digested slower and take more time to be processed. **This means that you're less likely to have blood sugar spikes, but stay full longer.**

- Not eating enough carbohydrates affects your mood. You may have noticed bodybuilders and others on high protein, low carb diets who are irritable and angry. This is often due to not getting enough carbohydrates.

How can you eat more whole grains?
The first step is to ensure all the grain and bread products you use are whole grains.

Here are a few ideas:

- You can start your day with whole grain wheat toast and oatmeal. Whole grain cereals taste delicious and help you feel fuller in the morning.

- Snack on whole grain crackers during the day or add quinoa chips to your routine.

- Another option is to ensure your pasta is always whole wheat.

- **Popcorn is a smart choice because it's considered whole grain.** Avoid drenching it in butter though, as that ruins the health benefits.

- When you make dinner, consider adding corn on the cob. Corn is a whole grain.

- Substitute brown or wild rice for the white version. Your family may actually enjoy the rich taste.

"Whole foods like grains and beans release their sugar very, very slowly because of the fiber in them, and they don't give you a sugar rush. They feed your cells as needed, and as a result, you have loads of stable energy that powers you through the day."

- Kathy Freston Day

ADD MORE BEETS

How often do you eat beets? The answer is probably not often, if at all.

Sadly, by skipping beets, you're missing out on many important nutrients that can affect your emotional wellbeing.

Beets are red root vegetables that have high levels of folate. This vitamin is essential for your brain and affects your mood. They also have phytonutrients known as betalains that are hard to find in other places.

Discover more about this surprising vegetable:

1. **Beets have B vitamin folate.** Folate is an essential vitamin that is part of beets. You need B vitamin folate because it can affect your mood, memory, and thinking abilities.

   - **When you have more folate in your body, research shows that you're more likely to be in a positive mood.** In addition, the risk of clinical depression decreases with more folate.

2. **Beets contain betaine.** Betaine is an amino acid that is used by the body to make SAM-e. You may have seen SAM-e being sold as a supplement in stores. However, your body can also make it, and some medical experts consider it a natural antidepressant.

3. **Beets also have betalains.** These substances are phytonutrients and have strong antioxidant and anti-inflammatory properties. The more antioxidant and anti-inflammatory nutrients you get, the healthier your brain becomes.

How do you eat more beets? Here are a few ways:

- Remember to get rid of the outer skin first and wash them thoroughly before cooking. It's also important to keep in mind that they can stain things red, including your stool. So just be mindful of that a day or two after you eat beets.

- Beets can be eaten raw. Try adding salt, pepper, and herbs to counteract the earthy flavor.

- Roast beets with other vegetables.

- Add them to salads and soups. Consider making a beet salad with cheese such as Feta cheese.

- You can make pickled beets at home. After boiling the beets, pour vinegar over the slices and store them in a clean jar. It takes about three days for them to be ready.

- Coleslaw isn't limited to cabbage. Beets add a beautiful red color and make the dish unique.

- Classic borscht soup can also be dressed up with beets.

- Consider using beets as a topping for pizza. Small slices of cooked beets go well with cheese and tomato sauce.

Beets are a fun and colorful addition to your diet. Not only will you get more folate and B vitamins, but you'll also feel better emotionally.

"The beet is the most intense of vegetables. The radish, admittedly, is more feverish, but the fire of the radish is a cold fire, the fire of discontent not of passion. Tomatoes are lusty enough, yet there runs through tomatoes an undercurrent of frivolity. The beet is the ancient ancestor of the autumn moon. . ."

- Tom Robbins

EAT WILD SALMON

Wild salmon has been the focus of several intriguing studies. Fish are a big part of the Mediterranean diet and other healthy diets around the world.

Salmon, particularly the wild variety, has multiple health benefits, including:

1. **Wild is better than farmed.** Wild salmon has fewer calories, half the fat, more calcium, more iron, more potassium, and more zinc than farmed salmon.

   - Studies show that farmed salmon doesn't have the same diet as wild fish. This ultimately affects the total number of nutrients you receive.

- In many stores around the globe, farmed salmon is more commonly available. If you're unsure, just ask the staff about where the fish is from.

- Although the wild version is more expensive, when given the choice, choose wild.

2. **Nutrients.** Wild salmon is packed with many nutrients for your body and brain, and these nutrients are essential for your emotional wellbeing. Salmon has omega-3s, zinc, magnesium, calcium, iron, and phosphorus.

   - **Research shows that eating more salmon decreases the risk of depression.** Study participants who had diets filled with salmon were also less likely to suffer from bipolar disorder and seasonal affective disorder.

Consider these tips to add more salmon into your diet:

- Sauté a fillet of salmon. You can do it in a skillet or pan with oil or butter.

- Poach salmon.

- Broiling, roasting, and searing are all good methods for the oven.

- Try cooking salmon wrapped in parchment paper. This allows you to seal in the flavor and add herbs directly on top. Some recipes also add vegetables to the parchment package for an all-in-one meal.

- One unusual way to cook salmon is inside fig leaves. You place the salmon on the leaves and bake them in the oven. The leaves help keep the fish moist.

- Sushi is also an option for getting more salmon in your diet.

Wild salmon is a great addition to your diet that's packed with many important nutrients. We recommend eating salmon at least once a week.

"I hate going out for lunch during a workday because it slows down my pace and ruins my rhythm. I prefer to eat at my desk. Actually, I wander around the design studio with a plate in my hand as I dine on, for example, salmon sashimi and a salad of tomatoes and mozzarella. I often have a bit of dark chocolate after lunch."

- Tom Ford

EAT A VARIETY OF FOODS

One important part of a healthy diet for emotional wellbeing is variety. How much variety is currently part of your diet? Do you eat the same food all the time? Doesn't that get boring?

Variety is the key to ensuring you get enough nutritional support to uplift your emotions.

Variety also helps you stay interested in your meals and encourages you to experiment with new foods. Keeping things interesting and different helps your brain stay active, so your mood is better. Your brain responds well to learning new things, and new food has a positive impact.

Plus, when you eat the same thing every day, you can get bored and this boredom can overflow into other parts of your life.

Remember to keep your plate colorful! You'll soon find that you enjoy eating new foods and colorful meals.

"Follow your dreams, work hard, practice and persevere. Make sure you eat a variety of foods, get plenty of exercise and maintain a healthy lifestyle."

- Sasha Cohen

FOCUS ON ORGANIC FOODS

One of the key ways to boost your wellbeing and increase happiness seems to be tied to organic foods.

Several studies have found that organic foods have higher levels of nutrients.

You need these nutrients such as vitamins and minerals for brain health and mood stability, so getting more of them is essential.

Consider these facts:

1. **Organic foods tend to have more nutritional value.**

- Organic foods are often grown differently compared to non-organic ones. In addition, many organic foods are grown from heirloom seeds which grow into plants that have more nutrients.

- Moreover, organic foods are grown without harmful pesticides that can affect your body.

2. **Pesticides and herbicides may be dangerous.** Several studies have found that many pesticides and herbicides are neurotoxins. Neurotoxins can harm your brain and body.

  - They may affect your mood and increase the risk of depression. They may interfere with the natural processes in your body that create happiness.

3. **Avoid the dirty dozen.** The dirty dozen are fruits and veggies that are most affected by pesticides and herbicides.

- For example, one study found that a small sample of strawberries had 20 different pesticides. Another study found that 98 percent of the dirty dozen fruits and vegetables had at least one pesticide residue left on them.

- **The current list of dirty dozen foods includes:**

  - Spinach
  - Strawberries
  - Nectarines

- Potatoes
- Apples
- Peaches
- Celery
- Grapes
- Cherries
- Pears
- Tomatoes
- Sweet bell peppers

- **Spinach** appears to be affected the most among the dirty dozen. It seems to have the highest residues of pesticides.

- It's important to note that the dirty dozen list gets updated regularly by environmental agencies and groups. The amount of pesticides used by food manufacturers can vary over time.

Organic foods are a vital part of a healthy diet that focuses on emotional wellbeing. They can affect your body, mind, and mood. They can influence how you feel long-term and may have an enormous impact on your wellbeing.

"If you can't afford organic food and are unable to grow your own, it's crucial to wash all inorganic produce very carefully to minimize the toxins you consume.

Soak everything for 20 minutes in water with vinegar and salt or water with fresh lemon juice and salt."

- Suzanne Somers

FINAL THOUGHTS

What you put on your plate can make a big difference in how you feel and act. Your diet can affect your mood and happiness levels.

From breakfast to late-night snacks, every morsel of food can either work to uplift you or hurt your mood and feelings.

There is a strong link between the food you eat and how you feel. Your brain relies on the nutrients from food just like your body, so the fuel you use to keep moving during the day also affects your mind.

From adding more blueberries to cooking with chili peppers, you can easily make adjustments to your diet that will benefit you. Focus on food that is organic, natural and plant-based.

Consider how you can add these foods to your meals throughout the day, and adjust recipes as you go. Soon, you'll be able to plan healthy meals ahead of time that are filled with nutrients that naturally boost your mood.

Start making these changes to your diet today. You'll be glad you did!

"Foods high in bad fats, sugar and chemicals are directly linked to many negative emotions, whereas whole, natural foods rich in nutrients – foods such as fruits, vegetables, grains and legumes – contribute to greater energy and positive emotions."

- Marilu Henner